HOW TO MAKE NATURAL FACE MASKS

DR MIRIAM KINAI

ISBN: 149271593X

ISBN-13: 978-1492715931

CONTENTS

DR MIRIAM KINAI

1

EQUIPMENT

Mixing bowl

Stirring spoon

Wide mouthed jar with tight fitting lid

*****

2

INGREDIENTS

1 tablespoon cosmetic clay like white or yellow kaolin clay

1 tablespoon powdered herbs like chamomile or lavender flowers

3 drops essential oils like lavender or tea tree essential oils

2 tablespoons wetting agent like water or aloe vera gel

1 teaspoon vitamin E oil (optional natural preservative with anti-oxidant properties)

* * * * *
, , , ,

3

INSTRUCTIONS

Mix the clay and the herbs with just enough wetting agent to form a paste

Add the essential oils as you stir

Add the vitamin E oil (if using)

Apply the paste to the face (avoiding the eye area) and let it dry

Wash it off with warm water and apply a moisturizer.

Tips

1. Make a large batch of the face mask but store the ingredients separately to extend their shelf life. For example you can mix the dry ingredients (cosmetic clay and powdered herbs) in a jar with a tight fitting lid. Then mix the wet ingredients (aloe vera gel, essential oils and vitamin E oil) in a dark colored jar and store the two jars in a cool place.

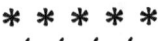

4

THERAPEUTIC FACE MASK RECIPES

Normal Skin Recipe

1 tablespoon cosmetic clays for normal skin like rose clay, yellow kaolin clay

1 tablespoon powdered herbs beneficial for normal skin like chamomile, lavender, rosemary, arnica, calendula flowers, comfrey

3 drops essential oils that can be used on normal skin like clary sage, eucalyptus, geranium, grapefruit, lavender, lemon, Roman chamomile, sweet orange, rosemary, peppermint, tea tree and ylang ylang.

2 tablespoons wetting agent that is perfect for normal skin like water, aloe vera gel, glycerine, rose water, honey, yogurt, milk, buttermilk, apple juice, lemon juice, pineapple puree, papaya puree

1 teaspoon vitamin E oil (optional natural preservative)

Follow the above Basic Face Mask Recipe Instructions.

7

Oily Skin Recipe

1 tablespoon cosmetic clays that are perfect for oily skin like Bentonite clay, French green clay, multani mitti clay, rhassoul clay, glacial clay

1 tablespoon powdered herbs or spices used to manage oily skin like turmeric powder, cinnamon powder, lavender flowers, rose petals, lemongrass, witch hazel or dried crushed neem leaves

3 drops essential oils used to manage oily skin and acne like tea tree, lemon, lavender, sandalwood

2 tablespoons wetting agent that is perfect for oily skin like aloe vera gel, honey, yogurt, milk (whole and skim), buttermilk, apple juice, lemon juice, pineapple puree, papaya puree

1 teaspoon vitamin E oil (optional natural preservative with anti-oxidant properties)

Follow the above Basic Face Mask Recipe Instructions.

***

Dry Skin Recipe

1 tablespoon cosmetic clays that are perfect for dry skin like rose clay, white kaolin clay, yellow kaolin clay, Moroccan red clay

1 tablespoon powdered ground herbs or spices used to manage dry skin like calendula flowers, chamomile flowers, lavender flowers, rosemary leaves, comfrey

3 drops essential oils used to manage dry skin like lavender, Roman chamomile, ylang ylang

2 tablespoons wetting agent that is perfect for dry skin like water, aloe vera gel, glycerine, rose water, honey, yogurt, milk (whole and skim), buttermilk

1 teaspoon vitamin E oil (optional natural preservative with anti-oxidant properties)

Follow the above Basic Face Mask Recipe Instructions.

Sensitive Skin Recipe

1 tablespoon cosmetic clays that can be used on sensitive skin like white kaolin clay, yellow kaolin clay

1 tablespoon powdered herbs or spices used to manage sensitive skin like calendula flowers, chamomile flowers, lavender flowers

3 drops essential oils

2 tablespoons wetting agent that is perfect for sensitive skin like water, aloe vera gel, glycerine, rose water, honey

1 teaspoon vitamin E oil (optional natural preservative with anti-oxidant properties)

Follow the above Basic Face Mask Recipe Instructions.

***

Mature Skin Recipe

1 tablespoon cosmetic clays that are good for mature skin like rose clay, white kaolin clay, yellow kaolin clay, Moroccan red clay

1 tablespoon powdered herbs or spices used to manage mature skin like calendula flowers, chamomile flowers, lavender flowers, green tea leaves, rose petals

3 drops essential oils used to manage mature skin like rose, geranium, clary sage, lavender essential oils

2 tablespoons wetting agent that is perfect for mature skin like strong green tea, water, aloe vera gel, glycerine, rose water, honey, yogurt, milk (whole and skim), buttermilk, apple juice

1 teaspoon vitamin E oil (optional natural preservative with anti-oxidant properties)

Follow the above Basic Face Mask Recipe Instructions.

Prematurely Aging Skin Recipe

1 tablespoon cosmetic clays that can be used on prematurely aging skin like rose clay, white kaolin clay, yellow kaolin clay, Moroccan red clay

1 tablespoon powdered herbs or spices used to manage prematurely aging skin like calendula flowers, chamomile flowers, lavender flowers, green tea leaves, rose petals

3 drops essential oils used to manage prematurely aging skin like patchouli, clary sage, rose, lavender, geranium

2 tablespoons wetting agent that is perfect for prematurely aging skin strong green tea, water, aloe vera gel, glycerine, rose water, honey, yogurt, milk (whole and skim), buttermilk, apple juice

1 teaspoon vitamin E oil (optional natural preservative with anti-oxidant properties)

Follow the above Basic Face Mask Recipe Instructions.

***

Eczema Recipe

1 tablespoon cosmetic clays that can be used on eczema prone skin like white kaolin clay, yellow kaolin clay

1 tablespoon powdered herbs used to manage eczema like calendula flowers, chamomile flowers

3 drops essential oils used to manage eczema like geranium, lavender, Roman chamomile and rosemary

2 tablespoons wetting agent that is perfect for eczema prone skin like water, aloe vera gel, honey, yogurt, milk (whole and skim)

1 teaspoon vitamin E oil (optional natural preservative with anti-oxidant properties)

Follow the above Basic Face Mask Recipe Instructions.

Psoriasis Recipe

1 tablespoon cosmetic clays that can be used on psoriasis prone skin like white kaolin clay, yellow kaolin clay

1 tablespoon powdered herbs used to manage psoriasis like chamomile flowers, calendula, chickweed, comfrey root

3 drops essential oils used to manage psoriasis like bergamot, tea tree, lavender, helichrysum, patchouli, rose, sandalwood

2 tablespoons wetting agent that is perfect for psoriasis prone skin like water, aloe vera gel, honey

1 teaspoon vitamin E oil (optional natural preservative)

Follow the above Basic Face Mask Recipe Instructions.

***

Coffee Lovers Recipe

1 tablespoon cosmetic clays like white kaolin clay or yellow kaolin clay

1 tablespoon powdered coffee

2 tablespoons brewed strong coffee

1 teaspoon vitamin E oil (optional natural preservative)

Follow the above Basic Face Mask Recipe Instructions.

***

Chocoholics Recipe

1 tablespoon cosmetic clays like white kaolin clay or yellow kaolin clay

1 tablespoon cocoa powder

2 tablespoons strong cocoa drink

1 teaspoon vitamin E oil (optional natural preservative

Follow the above Basic Face Mask Recipe Instructions.

5

ESSENTIAL OILS

Choose the aromatherapy essential oils you will use for your natural skincare products depending on your skin type and the condition that you want the product to manage.

Clary Sage Essential Oil

Clary Sage Essential Oil has an herbaceous scent. It can help relieve stress related tension, reduce irritability and help one relax. It is also used for the management of mature and acne prone skin.

Do not use it during pregnancy or if you are drinking alcohol or driving or if you have endometriosis, ovarian cysts, uterine cysts, breast cancer or you are at high risk for developing breast cancer as it may have an "estrogen-like" effect on the body.

***

Eucalyptus Essential Oil

Eucalyptus essential oil has an invigorating scent. It can help relieve stress related mental tension and mental exhaustion. It is also used in the management of joint aches and pains.

Do not use eucalyptus essential oil if you have epilepsy, high blood pressure or apply it near a baby's nostrils.

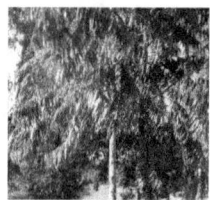

***

Geranium Essential Oil

Geranium Essential Oil has a fresh, minty rose scent. It can help relieve nervous tension and anxiety. It is also used in the management of eczema, cellulite as well as mature skin.

Avoid using it in pregnancy.

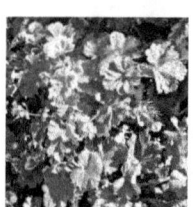

***

Grapefruit Essential Oil

Grapefruit essential oil has a refreshing, bitter-sweet scent. It can help relieve tension and release repressed emotions. It is also used in the management of cellulite.

Lavender Essential Oil

Lavender essential oil has a soothing, floral scent. It can help one relax and relieve stress related tension, sleeplessness, anxiety and depression. It is also used in the management of **acne, eczema and dry skin conditions.**

Do not use lavender essential oil in pregnancy, if you are breastfeeding, on young children as it may cause breast development in young boys and girls. Avoid it if you have low blood pressure as you may feel drowsy after using it.

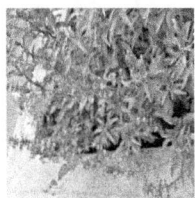

***

Lemon Essential Oil

Lemon essential oil has a clarifying fresh scent. It can help relieve mental tension, alleviate mental fatigue and increase concentration. It is also used in the management of acne and post acne dark skin spots.

Do not use it if skin will be exposed to sunlight or UV rays in the next 12-24 hours. Do not use it if you have low blood pressure or you are allergic to lemons.

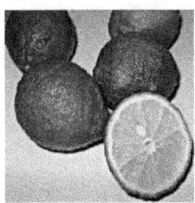

Lemongrass Essential Oil

Lemongrass essential oil has a vitalizing, lemony scent. It can help relieve tension and muscle aches. It is also used in the management of acne.

Do not use it if skin will be exposed to sunlight or UV rays in the next 12-24 hours.

***

Roman Chamomile Essential Oil

Roman chamomile essential oil has a sweet and fruity scent. It can help relieve stress related tension headaches. It is also used in the management of eczema, psoriasis and dry skin conditions.

Avoid using it in pregnancy and if you are allergic to ragweed.

***

Spearmint Essential Oil

Spearmint essential oil has a gently-energizing minty scent. It can help relieve mental tension and exhaustion. It is also used in the management of nausea.

***

Rose Essential Oil

Rose essential oil has a sweet and floral scent. It has mentally cheering properties and is used to relieve depression, sorrow and heartache. It is also useful for mature and prematurely aging skin.

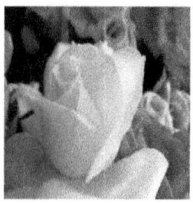

Rosemary Essential Oil

Rosemary Essential Oil has an uplifting and stimulating scent. It can help relieve mental exhaustion and feeling rundown. It is also used in the management of dry skin, eczema, muscle aches and joint pains.

Do not use rosemary essential oil if you are pregnant or have epilepsy or high blood pressure. Avoid using it if you have a fever or you want to sleep and in children under 5 years.

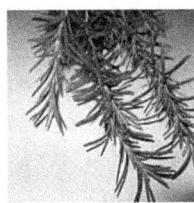

***

Sweet Orange Essential Oil

Sweet orange essential oil has a cheeringly, refreshing scent. It can help mange stress related tension. It is also used in the management of cellulite and common colds.

Do not use it if skin will be exposed to sunlight or UV rays in the next 12-24 hours.

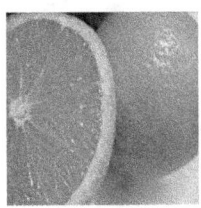

***

Peppermint Essential Oil

Peppermint essential oil has a head-clearing, refreshing scent. It can help relieve tension and fatigue. It is also used to manage flatulence.

Do not use peppermint essential oil in pregnancy, if breastfeeding, on children less than 5 years, if you have epilepsy or irregular heartbeats or cardiac fibrillation or high blood pressure and before using a sun bed or going to hot humid places.

***

Tea Tree Essential Oil

Tea tree essential oil has a purifying almost medicinal scent. It can help relieve tension and fatigue. It is also been used in the management of oily skin, acne and athlete's foot.

***

Ylang Ylang Essential Oil

Ylang ylang essential oil has a fragrantly floral scent. It can help relieve anxiety, tension and help one relax. It is also used as an aphrodisiac and in the management of dry skin conditions.

Do not use ylang ylang essential oil if you have low blood pressure or sensitive, damaged skin.

* * * * *

6

HERBS

Choose the herbs you will use for your natural skincare products depending on your skin type and the condition that you want the product to manage.

Aloe Vera

Aloe vera has anti-inflammatory properties and acts as a soothing balm for inflamed skin. It also stimulates cell regeneration and is vital for healing. Since it contains over 90% water, it is also an excellent moisturizer.

***

Arnica Flowers

Arnica flowers are believed to have anti-inflammatory properties and are used to relieve the pains of sprains, muscle aches and joint pains.

Do not use arnica if you are allergic to it, if pregnant or breastfeeding.

Calendula Flowers

Calendula flowers are used to manage dry, sensitive, mature, prematurely aging and normal skin types.

Calendula flowers also have antioxidant, anti-inflammatory and anti-infective properties. They are therefore also used to help wounds, minor cuts and bruises, small insect bites, first degree burns, mild sunburns and mild skin infections heal faster.

Calendula is also a soothing agent which reduces inflammation and it has been shown to prevent dermatitis or skin inflammation in breast cancer patients receiving radiation treatment.

Do not use calendula if you are allergic to it, allergic to daisy or aster family plants like ragweed and chrysanthemums, if pregnant or breastfeeding or trying to conceive. Avoid calendula preparations if you are taking sedatives, high blood pressure and diabetes medications.

***

Chamomile Flowers

Chamomile flowers are used to manage dry, sensitive, oily, mature, prematurely aging and normal skin types.

Chamomile flowers have anti-inflammatory activity and mild antiseptic properties. They are also soothing to the skin and help in eliminating blackheads by helping open up the pores.

Chamomile flowers also have mentally relaxing properties and are used to relieve anxiety and emotional stress as well as to relax tense muscles and relieve muscle spasms.

Do not use/ avoid chamomile if you are allergic to it, allergic to daisy or aster family plants such as ragweed and chrysanthemums, have asthma, are pregnant as it may cause miscarriage, if driving as it may cause drowsiness, if taking alcohol, for at least 2 weeks before surgery or dental procedures as it may cause bleeding. Do not use/avoid chamomile if you are taking blood thinners like warfarin (coumadin), clopidogrel (plavix) or aspirin as it may cause bleeding, sedatives, high blood pressure medications and diabetes medications.

Comfrey Leaves

Comfrey leaves are used to manage dry and normal skin types.

Comfrey leaves have anti-inflammatory, skin regenerative and antiseptic properties. They are also used to relieve muscle strains and ligament sprains.

Do not use/ avoid comfrey if you are allergic to it, on broken skin, on children, the elderly, if pregnant or breastfeeding, in liver disease, alcoholism and cancer. Do not use/ avoid comfrey if you are taking acetaminophen (panadol, tylenol). Do not use/ avoid comfrey if using herbs known to cause liver problems such as kava, valerian and skullcap.

***

Lavender Flowers

Lavender flowers are used to treat eczema and manage dry, sensitive, mature, prematurely aging, normal, oily and acne prone skin.

Lavender flowers have calming, analgesic, anti-inflammatory and skin regenerative properties. They are also used to manage stress, reduce anxiety and insomnia and relieve muscle and joint aches.

Do not use/ avoid lavender if you are allergic to it, on broken skin, if pregnant or breastfeeding, on young boys as it may cause male breast development. Do not use/ avoid lavender if you are taking sedatives, anti-anxiety medications such as lorazepam and narcotic analgesics such as morphine and oxycodone.

Rose Petals

Rose petals are used to manage oily, mature and prematurely aging skin.

Rose petals are also believed to have skin softening properties.

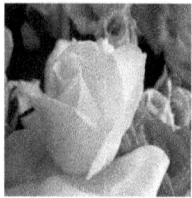

***

Rosemary Leaves

Rosemary leaves are used to manage dry and normal skin.

Rosemary leaves have antioxidant and antimicrobial properties. They are mentally stimulating and are used to reduce feelings of sadness or depression, increase mental concentration and relieve muscle pains and joint aches.

Do not use/ avoid rosemary if you are allergic to it, are breastfeeding or pregnant as it may cause miscarriages, are under 18 years old, have high blood pressure, peptic ulcers, ulcerative colitis or Crohn's disease. Do not use/avoid rosemary if you are taking blood thinners such as warfarin (coumadin), clopidogrel (plavix) or aspirin as it may cause bleeding, angiotensin converting enzyme (ACE) inhibitors such as captopril and lisinopril for high blood pressure, diuretics such as furosemide (lasix) and hydrochlorothiazide also used for high blood pressure treatment and medicines for diabetes medications as it may alter the blood sugar levels and lithium.

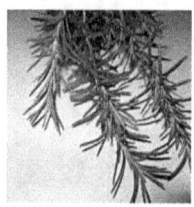

Sage

Sage contains vitamins A, B complex, C, E, K and the mineral calcium, copper and magnesium. It also has astringent properties which are perfect for oily skincare and hair care products. Sage has been show by some clinical trials to raise the mood and lower anxiety and it is therefore used to treat depression. It is also used to improve the memory. Sage also reduces excessive sweating and the hot flashes of menopause. It is also said to reduce the mood swings associated with menopause. It is also used to whiten teeth.

***

St John's Wort Flowers And Leaves

St John's Wort flowers and leaves have anti-depressant, anti-inflammatory, antiseptic properties. They are used to relieve mild depression, and manage mild eczema.

Do not use/ avoid St John's wort if you are allergic to it, have major or severe depression and bipolar disorder, are pregnant, breastfeeding or trying to get pregnant. Do not use/ avoid St John's wort if you are going to have surgery in five days, are taking digoxin for the heart, antiretroviral medicines used to treat HIV/ AIDS, if you are taking medications to treat depression as it could result in the dangerous serotonin syndrome. These antidepressant medications include serotonin reuptake inhibitors (SSRIs) such as citalopram, fluoxetine and sertraline, tricyclic antidepressants such as amitriptyline and imipramine, monoamine oxidase inhibitors (MAOIs) such as phenelzine and tranylcypromine.

***

Witch Hazel

Witch hazel is used to manage oily skin.

It is an astringent which tightens the pores and removes excessive oils. It also has healing properties.

* * * * *
, , , ,

7

SPICES

Choose the spices you will use for your natural skincare products depending on your skin type and the condition that you want the product to manage.

Cinnamon

Cinnamon is useful for managing acne and acne prone skin.

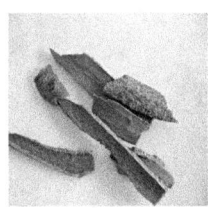

Cloves

Cloves have natural antibacterial and antiviral properties. Clove oil is also used to relieve toothaches.

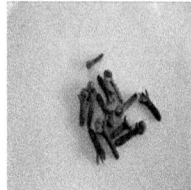

***

Turmeric

Turmeric is used to manage oily or acne prone skin.

Turmeric which is a potent antioxidant, also has antiseptic properties when it is applied to the skin.

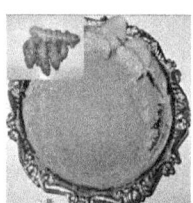

* * * * *

8

SKIN FOOD

Choose the food items you will use for your natural skincare products depending on your skin type and the condition that you want the product to manage.

Apples

Juiced or pureed apples are great for the skin because apples contain 85% water and vitamins A and C. These vitamins are potent antioxidants which protect the skin cells from the free radical damage that contributes to premature aging. Apples also contain malic acid which is great for exfoliating and removing dead cells from the skin's surface.

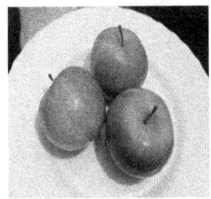

Beeswax

Beeswax helps seal in moisture and prevents the skin from drying. When used to make natural skin care products, it acts as an emulsifier.

***

Coffee

Coffee is an excellent exfoliant which removes the dead cells on the surface of the skin. It also contains the anti-inflammatory caffeic acid which is also said to increase skin's collagen production.

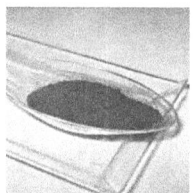

***

Honey

Honey has antiseptic activity which is useful for controlling infections and healing the skin. It is also a humectant which helps keep the skin moisturized. Honey also softens the skin. In addition, it is also a powerful antioxidant which is useful for preventing free radical damage to skin cells that causes premature aging.

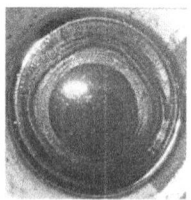

***

Lemon

Lemon contains natural acids which aid in exfoliation and lightening dark marks like acne scars. It can also be used as a toner for oily skin.

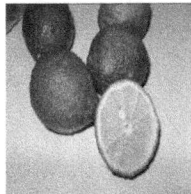

***

Milk

Milk regardless of whether it is whole, skimmed or buttermilk, contains lactic acid, which is an alpha hydroxy acid (AHA), that helps slough away the dead cells on the surface of the skin. In addition, milk products help the skin retain its moisture as they gently exfoliate it.

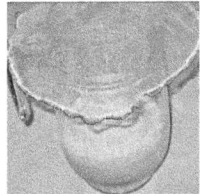

***

Neem

Neem is an effective skin antiseptic which kills bacteria and soothes inflammation without further irritating the skin.

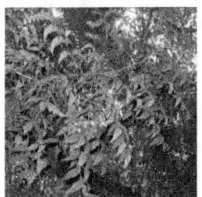

Papaya or Pawpaw

Papaya or pawpaw contains papain which is a natural enzyme that removes the dead cells from the surface of the skin without irritating it.

In addition, papaya also contains the anti-oxidant vitamins A, C and E which protect the skin from free radical cell damage.

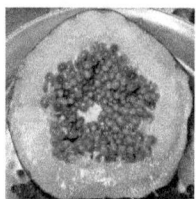

***

Pineapple

Pineapple has natural enzymes which remove the dead cells on the surface of the skin without causing irritation.

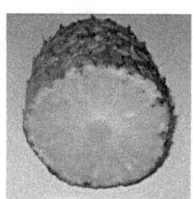

***

Yoghurt

Yogurt contains a natural acid called lactic acid which gently exfoliate the skin while moisturizing it.

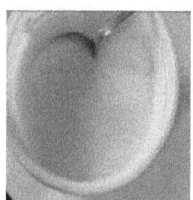

* * * * *
' ' ' '

9

NATURAL CLAYS

Choose the natural cosmetic clays you will use for your all natural skin care products depending on your skin type and the condition that you want the product to manage.

Bentonite Clay

Bentonite clay, which is also called Montmorillonite, is very useful for making skin care products for oily skin. It is particularly effective for making natural masks since it acts as a deep cleansing agent drawing out the excess oil from the skin pores.

French Green Clay

French green clay, which is also called sea clay, is one of the most commonly used cosmetic clays. This natural exfoliant is rich in minerals and nutrients. When used to make products for oily skin, it also doubles up as a deep cleansing agent since it is able to draw out the excess oil from the skin pores.

Glacial Clay

Glacial clay is obtained from a prehistoric formation in Canada. It is used to draw out oil from the skin especially in oily skin types.

***

Moroccan Red Clay

Moroccan red clay is used to make skin care products for dry skin since it cleanses the skin and moisturizes it.

***

Rhassoul Clay

Rhassoul clay is a light brown clay from Morocco. It is used to make products for oily skin types since it draws the excess oil from the skin.

***

Rose Clay

Rose clay is a mild-medium weight kaolin clay that cleanses the skin and improves its circulation. It is perfect for normal to dry skin.

***

White Kaolin Clay

White kaolin clay, which is also known as China clay or white clay, is used to make sensitive skin and dry skin types.

***

Yellow Kaolin Clay

Yellow kaolin clay is a mild clay that is perfect for making masks for normal skin types. This gentle exfoliant and cleanser which also stimulates the skin's blood supply is suitable for sensitive skin.

* * * * *

10

NATURAL PRESERVATIVES

Natural preservatives used to make skin care products include:

Rosemary Oleoresin

Rosemary oleoresin, which is also known as ROE, is a natural antioxidant extracted from the rosemary herb. It contains carnosic acid which extends the shelf life of homemade products by reducing the oxidation of their natural ingredients.

***

Vitamin E Oil

Vitamin E oil which usually comes as a mixture of tocopherols is natural antioxidant extracted from vegetable oils. Vitamin E oil is heat stable and can be used to extend the shelf life of products which do not contain water.

Grapefruit Seed Extract

Grapefruit seed extract is rich in vitamins C and E which are natural antioxidants. It is also able to kill or inhibit the growth of bacteria and fungi. It therefore functions both as a broad spectrum preservative and as an antioxidant.

###

ABOUT THE AUTHOR

Dr. Miriam Kinai is a medical doctor and a certified clinical aromatherapy practitioner.

You can visit her blog at http://www.MyBlogBookClub.com or follow her on twitter at http://twitter.com/AlmasiHealth

Email enquiries to almasihealthcare@yahoo.com with BOOKS as your subject.

HOW TO MAKE NATURAL SKIN CARE PRODUCTS SERIES

Books in this series include:

* How to Make Natural Anti-Wrinkle Creams and Anti-Aging Serums

* How to Make Natural Bath and Body Oils

* How to Make Natural Bath Bombs

* How to Make Natural Bath Cookies

* How to Make Natural Bath Melts

* How to Make Natural Bath Milks

* How to Make Natural Bath Salts

* How to Make Natural Bath Teas

* How to Make Natural Body Butters

* How to Make Natural Body Lotions

* How to Make Natural Body Scrubs

* How to Make Natural Body Wash

* How to Make Natural Cold Cream

* How to Make Natural Face Cleansers

* How to Make Natural Face Masks

* How to Make Natural Face Scrubs

* How to Make Natural Healing Balms

* How to Make Natural Herb Infused Oils

* How to Make Natural Massage Bars

HOW TO MAKE NATURAL FACE MASKS

* How to Make Natural Soap

* How to Make Natural Solid and Liquid Castile Soap

* How to Make Natural Solid and Liquid Perfumes

* How to Make Natural Sunscreen Lotions

* How to Make Natural Toothpaste, Tooth Whitening Powder and Mouthwash

* How to Make Ubtan Powder

*****

SIMPLIFIED MEDICINE

Simplified Medicine uses plain and easy to understand English to teach you about the causes, risk factors, symptoms, tests, treatment, prognosis and prevention of numerous diseases like:

* Bile Duct Cancer

* Osteosarcoma (Bone Cancer)

* Throat Cancer

* Congestive Heart Failure

* Legionnaire's Disease

* West Nile Virus

* Cryptosporidiosis

* Cyclospora

* Polymyalgia Rheumatica

* Sarcoidosis

* Alcoholic liver cirrhosis

* Dry Drowning

* Prosopagnosia

*****

HERBS AND SPICES FOR THE COOK, HEALER AND BEAUTICIAN

Herbs and Spices for the Cook, Healer and Beautician uses color pictures and clear explanations to teach you about more than 70 healing herbs and spices.

You will learn about their:

* Therapeutic (healing) uses

* Drug interactions

* Contraindications (when not to use them)

* Cooking tips

* Beauty tips

*****

CHRISTIAN LIFE COACHING HANDBOOK

Christian Life Coaching Handbook offers a Biblical approach to managing different aspects of life.

You will learn:

* Christian anger management

* Christian conflict resolution

* Christian depression treatment

* Christian goal setting

* Christian marital stress management

* Christian stress management

* How to assert yourself

* How to defeat fear

* How to love yourself

* How to overcome shyness

* How to resist temptation

* How to stop being a people pleaser

*****

CHRISTIAN SPIRITUAL WARFARE

Christian Spiritual Warfare teaches you the awesome Bible verses you can use as spiritual warfare prayers, Christian affirmations and in your Christian meditation sessions as you fight your spiritual battles.

You will learn how to fight for the following with Bible verses:

* Marriage * Children * Health

* Christian Faith * Christian Ministry

* Country

* Finances * Job * Business

* Peace of Mind * Restoration * Self Esteem * Self Love

You will also learn how to fight against the following with Bible verses:

* Addiction * Temptation

* Being Single * Infertility

* Opposition * Oppression

* Worry * Fear

* Feelings of Condemnation * Confusion

* Danger * Death * Despair * Discouragement

* Impatience * Insomnia * Laziness * Loneliness

* Poverty * Pride * Sadness

* Vengeance * Weakness

* A Foul Mouth * Lying

*****

DARK SKIN DERMATOLOGY COLOR ATLAS

Dark Skin Dermatology Color Atlas is filled with clear explanations and color photos of skin, hair, and nail diseases affecting people with skin of color or Fitzpatrick skin types IV, V, and VI.

Topics covered include Acne Vulgaris, Alopecia Areata, Anal Warts, Angioedema, Aphthous Ulcers, Atopic Dermatitis, Blastomycosis, Blister Beetle Dermatitis or Nairobi Fly Dermatitis, Cellulitis, Chronic Ulcers, Confetti Hypopigmentation, Cutaneous T Cell Lymphoma, Cutaneous Tuberculosis, Dermatitis Artefacta, Erythema Nodosum,

Exfoliative Erythroderma, Gianotti Crosti Syndrome, Hand Dermatitis, Hemangioma, Herpes Zoster, Ichthyosis, Ingrown Toenails, Irritant Contact Dermatitis, Kaposi Sarcoma, Keloids, Keratoderma Blenorrhagica, Klippel Trenaunay Weber Syndrome, Leishmaniasis, Leprosy, Leukonychia, Lichen Nitidus, Lichen Planus,

Lichenoid Drug Eruption, Linear Epidermal Nevus, Linear IgA Dermatosis (LAD), Lipodermatosclerosis, Lymphangioma Circumscriptum, Miliaria, Molluscum Contagiosum, Neurofibromatosis, Nickel Dermatitis, Onychomadesis, Onychomycosis, Palmoplantar Eccrine Hidradenitis, Papular Pruritic Eruption (PPE), Paronychia, Pellagra, Pemphigus Foliaceous,

Pemphigus Vulgaris, Piebaldism, Pityriasis Rosea, Pityriasis Rubra Pilaris, Plantar Hyperkeratosis, Plantar Warts, Poikiloderma, Postinflammatory Hyperpigmentation and Hypopigmentation, Post Topical Steroids Hypopigmentation, Psoriasis, Pyogenic Granuloma or Lobular Capillary Hemangioma, Scabies, Seborrheic Dermatitis, Steven Johnson Syndrome (SJS) and Toxic Epidermal Necrolysis (TEN),

Sunburn, Systemic Sclerosis, Tinea Capitis, Tinea Pedis, Tinea Versicolor, Traction Alopecia, Urticaria, Vasculitis, Vitiligo, and Xanthelasma.

*****

www.ingramcontent.com/pod-product-compliance
Lightning Source LLC
Chambersburg PA
CBHW070840290526
45795CB00002B/934